Leader of the Band

The Story of a Four-time Cancer Survivor

By Nick Pozza
Edited by Melanie Burt

Epigraph Books
Rhinebeck, New York

Leader of the Band © 2015 by Nick Pozza

Contact the publisher for information.

Printed in the United States of America

Book design by Colin Rolfe

Cover design by David Perry

Library of Congress Control Number: 2015945276

ISBN: 978-1-936940-60-8

Epigraph Books
22 East Market Street, Suite 304
Rhinebeck, NY 12572
www.epigraphps.com

Dedicated to my very supportive family,
oncology doctors and their staff,
and cancer survivors everywhere

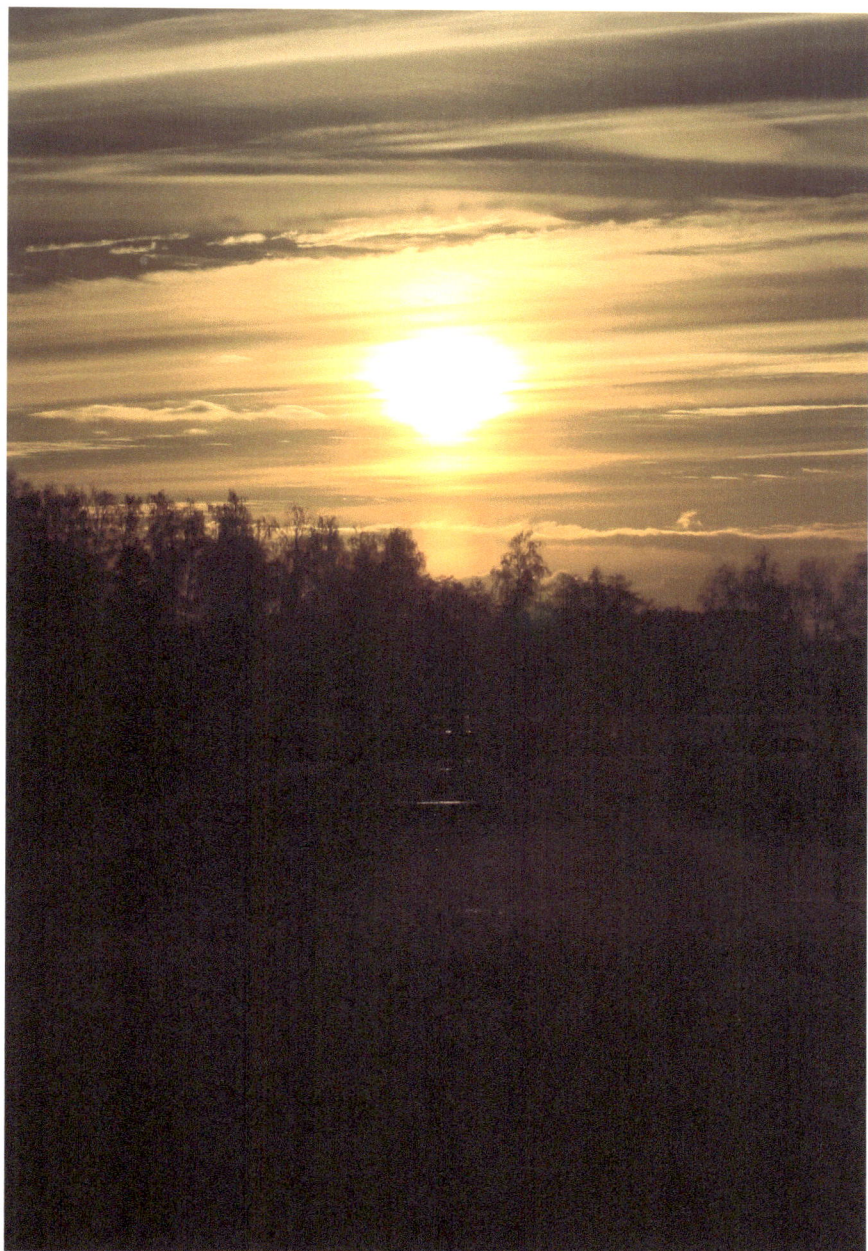

Sunrise
A New Beginning

I ought to sell my DNA. I've beat cancer four times and I'll beat it again if I have to. But let's hope it doesn't come to that. Those who know me best won't readily believe that I, Nick Pozza, willingly sat down and wrote about my experience with cancer—or my experience with anything for that matter. I can't say I blame them because, as my wife would tell you, I've never picked up a book or put pen to paper voluntarily in my 77 years. It wasn't until I had beaten cancer for the fourth time that I considered the possibility that others could take some solace from my story. A life handed back to me four times.

In August of 2012, I experienced shortness of breath. A chest x-ray revealed a spot on my lung which was classified as stage 3 lung cancer. My life was now one long string of doctors' appointments and treatments. It was hard to tell where one ended and another began. A PET scan found small peripheral lesions—evidence of more cancer. It was then that an MRI was scheduled to determine if the cancer had spread to my brain, but I could have told them nothing gets through this brain. Now I can boast to my wife such a characteristic is in fact a good thing. (Somewhere she's rolling her eyes right now.) Since the cancer was found to be localized to the lung, I could be scheduled for treatment. I was warned I would not survive surgery due to the location and size of the tumor and therefore, my only option was to combine radiation and chemotherapy.

Prior to my doctor taking a biopsy from my affected lung, I had to go through several breathing tests and exercises. This took the better part of the day. I had to breathe for the attending nurse. Then, I had to go in a chamber and perform more controlled breathing exercises. My blood pressure was monitored while this part of the test was performed. Once this was completed, my doctor could take the biopsy. I was sedated during that procedure. When I woke up, I remember asking the doctor when he was going to do it...he smiled and said that it was already done! Obviously, whatever they gave me worked pretty well! After many consultations with all of the doctors involved, my treatment was scheduled.

From October into November I endured radiation treatments Monday through Friday —a total of 30—at the Dyson Center. Once a week chemotherapy treatments were also scheduled, each of which lasted approximately 5 hours. I sat in a large room with other people also undergoing various infusion treatments. Some napped, some watched TV or read. Some of us chatted to pass the time. Five hours equals a lot of time with one's thoughts. It's strange how the mind wanders- never organized or chronological, and rarely to a momentous occasion. Rather, it jumps from one small exchange or happenstance to the next.

At one point I thought back to a job I had taken after retirement (I was not good at "relaxing and taking it easy"). Doing accounting work for a local business, I was also responsible for feeding the barnyard cats each morning. Such is the rural life outside of Poughkeepsie, New York. The cats knew I represented their morning meal and would come to greet me right away. One morning they did not come. Some chickens came instead. It seemed I was surrounded, strange as that sounds. As I started to chase them off, a rooster came out of nowhere and literally attacked me. I fell to the ground, at which point my right hand landed on a piece of angle iron, resulting in eight stitches and a tetanus shot. I couldn't help but laugh. Here I was fighting cancer for the fourth time and yet the record, in its merciless tally of truth, did remind me that I'd been bested by chickens.

I know that most people who choose to read my account are those who are fighting cancer or those who are fighting alongside. Accept the support of others. Keep your family close. Your very survival depends on this. I was never alone. Either my son or daughter accompanied me to every doctor's appointment, every treatment, every follow-up, and every consultation. My wife stayed home caring for our three grandchildren so our children could be with me. My daughter went online and found a prescription assistance program to help cover costs we couldn't. Both my children work for the New York State Police and have very understanding, compassionate, and supportive supervisors which allowed them the freedom to take time off whenever I needed them. Thank you New York State Police!

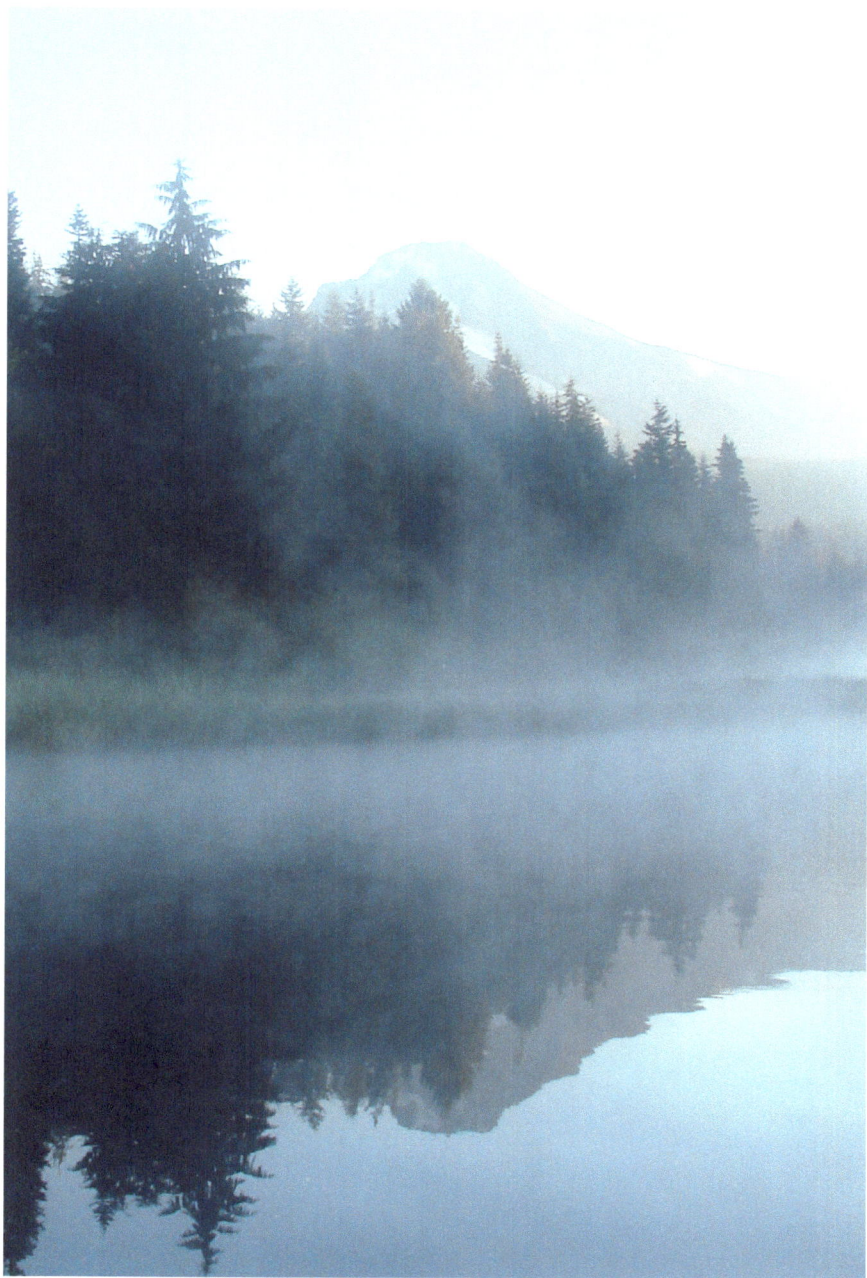

Peace and Tranquility

Support for my personal fight came from many different corners. From employees of the grocery store I go to every week to members of a local church that my children belong to. Everyone sent positive wishes and prayed on my behalf. The local Prayer Shawl Ministry sent my wife a prayer shawl crocheted by a member of the congregation and blessed by the pastor. As you can see, it takes a village to beat cancer. No one beats it alone. No one should have to.

Not only have I beaten cancer, but I have been on the front lines of medical treatments and technologies. In December of 1997 I took advantage of a free screening for prostate cancer. That screening led me to a urologist who found my PSA (prostate specific antigen) to be elevated. PSA, produced by the prostate, can detect prostate cancer or prostate abnormalities. It was cancer. I had three options. One—remove the prostate, two—delay treatment and schedule more tests, or three—have radiation seeds implanted into my prostate. My doctor and I chose curtain number three.

In January 1998, one hundred and one seeds were implanted. The timing of this treatment was tricky. With radiation seed implants, I could not be within six feet of pregnant women or young children, due to the high radiation levels, for the next six to seven months. Shortly after that procedure I recall entering a restaurant and having to carefully choose the location of my table because there were several young children there. Any time I was headed to a store I had to be conscious of who was around me. At this time, my son and daughter-in-law were expecting their first child. I remember a family dinner when we got the yardstick out and set up a tray table precisely six feet away from me for her to "enjoy" her meal at.

We laugh about it now, but keeping my distance was a strain on us all. We are a close family both emotionally and geographically. Having to keep my distance made me appreciate the time I get to spend with my immediate family on a daily basis. Most families don't enjoy that luxury. I believe if we tightened our radius by just a few miles, we could have ourselves a compound!

I was scheduled for many oncology appointments subsequent to the seed implants in order to ensure that infection did not set in. At each appointment I was asked to provide a urine sample. The first sample was particularly memorable because we did not expect it to come out green. A glow-in-the-dark, science fiction, you're-a-mean-one-Mister-Grinch shade of green. This was, to say the least, alarming to my nurse and caused quite the stir among the staff. As is often the case when one's urine turns green, it was all much ado about nothing. My doctor assured everyone that the incongruous hue was the result of the seeds. After-all, it was radiation, but since I was the first in my community to receive this treatment, a learning curve was to be expected.

I'm no stranger to cancer. I'm no stranger to loss. They touched my life long before my diagnosis. I grew up in a small, very rural town in Dutchess County - north of New York City. Both my parents came from Italy and only spoke Italian at the time. Naturally, I spoke primarily Italian prior to starting school. I depended on my sisters for help with my homework, as well as out in the world. I had an older brother who died at the age of nine from an ear infection. Due to the brutal New York winter, a doctor could not reach our home, and thus we had no access to medication. I was three at the time. I feel lucky to be living in this time and place where such tragedies are now practically unheard of. I am grateful for the medical and technological advances available to me that my brother was not privy to.

Both my mother and father died of cancer as well as my two older sisters. My mother died at age seventy-eight, my father at sixty-seven. My sisters succumbed at ages sixty-seven and seventy-six. Many of my aunts, uncles, and cousins have also died of cancer on both sides of my family. Now there is just myself and my younger sister who remain. Despite my family history, I never thought I would be diagnosed with cancer. Probably the result of my stubborn Italian ways. I can just feel the breeze coming from the zealous nods of my family's heads. The same stubbornness that kept me from believing I would ever have cancer was exactly what I needed to fight it, especially when I was fighting two types of cancer at one time.

In February of 1998, as I was battling prostate cancer (re: "the seeds"), I was also diagnosed with melanoma. During a semiannual check-up with my dermatologist, a spot was found on my back that looked like a blackhead. The biopsy revealed skin cancer. Three weeks later, this small spot had spread approximately eight inches. To make a short story even shorter, the melanoma was surgically removed and my back has been cancer-free since.

It should be of no surprise to the reader at this point that the melanoma found on my back in 1998 was not my first experience with skin cancer. In 1985, I saw a dermatologist out of concern for a spot on my nose. At first, a laser was used to remove the spot, but it re-appeared a few months later. It was another dermatologist who diagnosed the melanoma which was then treated with several rounds of micro surgery. To this day, my Italian nose is cancer free and remains my best feature. (Refer to back cover.)

As you can tell, I just don't know when to give up. Sometimes a blessing, sometimes a curse, but you'll have to agree, it works for me most of the time. As I said, it's strange how the mind works. Again, as I waited for the chemo and radiation to do their best (and their worst), I recalled another small accident I had.

Just months after the chicken incident I spoke of earlier, I had a run-in with my garage door. You see, our house, built in 1935, has a heavy wooden garage door held together with carriage bolts. As I was closing it, I didn't release my hand and so my thumb got caught between a bolt and the handle. Consequently, a chunk of my thumb was ripped clear off. In fact half my thumb print was gone. After driving myself to the ER to get it looked at, I was referred to a plastic surgeon for graphing. I was subsequently warned it was likely I would be left with permanent nerve damage. Again, I beat the odds. My thumb is in intact and nerve-damage free. I don't listen much to odds. Why should I? A chunk of my thumb is probably still stuck in the door for all I know. I didn't bother to look because I am always too busy moving on, too busy to look back, and of course too busy driving myself to the hospital.

Okay, so I'm a stubborn fellow as my family and friends can tell you. I could go on about that, as could those around me, but that would be fodder for another book. I want to mention a time in my life from where I draw strength, and a gift I received during that time which came to mean more to me than I could have ever known at the time.

In 1975 my twelve year old son, who was (and still is) a drummer, came to me with hopes of joining a marching band. There were none in our area, so I told him we couldn't drive that far. He simply asked me to start one in our own hometown. That's how kids think. That's how we should all think. Truth is I couldn't think of a reason not to. I remember my wife said, "Nick, are you crazy?" and to that I replied, "No, give me the phone!". I immediately called friends to help get it all started. The parents of some of my son's musician friends and a music teacher at a local high school pitched in. Although my son was just twelve, he was also a great help with ideas and suggestions.

With simple home-made fliers, we advertised the formation of the band, and were looking for youths to join. I arranged to use a local elementary school facility for practice—26 members signed up that first night. We started off slow with just one song that we played on the sidewalk in front of a local bank. We played "Aquarius" over and over again for two hours. If those bank tellers didn't know that song going into work, they sure knew it coming out. Gradually, we built a name for ourselves with more and more youths signing up and thankfully more and more songs in our repertoire. Ultimately, we reached a membership of 110.

We were a "junior marching band" made up of local children ages 10 through 18. Our colors of choice were lime green and white so we would stand out as we marched down the street. You could see "The Green Machine" coming a mile away ! I can tell you that my wife knows a thing or two about lime green. She ironed and fitted lime green pants, lime green flags, lime green cumber bunds, neck scarves, sashes and bags. This was done with the help of talented local seamstresses, most of whom were parents of our band members. The uniforms were handmade and each spring were tailored to fit every member. No internet or catalog orders here! If there was something lime-green floating around, no youth between the ages of 10 and 18 was safe. For all I know, there may be the occasional lime green piece of apparel in the local consignment shops. If you have happened across any, you're welcome. You know what they say- lime green is the new black. Or at least that's what you say if you were a member of the band.

Over the dozen or so years (and hundreds of members) we marched in numerous parades, including the Elks Convention Parade, played in pre-game and half-time shows at Yankee Stadium, and even played a half-time show for the Giants/Cowboys game at Giant Stadium. Those children worked hard and it showed in both the numerous awards, many miles on their feet and smiles on their faces! I wonder how many miles I have walked? They say exercise is good for you.

Now for the gift I mentioned earlier. One of the band members, a girl in her mid teens at the time, wrote a set of eight poems and stories for me. Her words changed me somehow. They inspired a more optimistic point of view, which I still enjoy to this day. I don't know if it was the poems alone or the fact they came from someone so young that made the difference. In any case, I have included one of them here to honor the comfort and perspective it has afforded me through the years.

"The room was dark, lit only by the reddish orange glow of the blazing fire roaring in the stone fireplace. The stones of the hearth, black freckled with soot, seemed to radiate heat as thick in the air as the falling January snow blowing in the wind outside the frost covered window. An oil lamp, stained from years of reliable service, stood on a wooden, oak carved bed stand. Once thick woolen rugs now comfortably worn to a soft grassy texture, has streaks of light cast upon it by the fire. The large oaken bed has sheer lace covering its four high posters and canopy. The exposed floor showed years of wear making it as soft as the rugs scattered on it. The dark corners were not threatening, but inviting with the deep cushioned, high-back chairs nestled there. Ghosts from the past ran rapidly, but silently around, lending an air of comfort and romance to the primeval cathedral windows. Tapestries covered grey walls, bringing to them scenes of valley and mountain, river and ocean. The bed, draped in goose down. The bed itself was cozy as if made of the most delicate cloud from a fairytale land. The solid door was carved as were the bed stand and bed, and when it closed, it did so with the sound of a boulder fitting snugly into the stony cave of a mystical shroud. Inside was a place of consolation, beauty, rest, and pure passion. This room, nestled in a small stone home, back in the high trees of a far-away forest, is the room I often dream of and see myself cuddled up in cozy warmth, protected from the world. Someday I will find this room. It may be in an apartment in a busy city, in a townhouse in some suburban town, but I know I will find it because it exists. If I should never ascertain it, then it will always be in my mind for me to visit when I'm lonely or cold."

Remarkably, she left a note on one of the poems which read, "Someday this might be worth something." I led the band for 14 years, at which point I decided it was time for me to retire. The band disbanded shortly after, but the bonds my family and I forged with some of the members have remained strong over the years. They are as close as family to this day.

As you can see, I place a great deal of emphasis on this part of my life. I take strength from my accomplishments and surround myself with those who have made the good times in fact, the good times.

Segue to my wife, who has provided the comfort and stability I have depended on for 55 years, and who has given me a family that surrounds me every day of my life. We met at a fireman's ball near my hometown. She had come with her boyfriend, but that didn't bother me any. In fact, he and I were friends and he was the one who introduced us.

Further proof that life imitates art, our first dance was to the Tennessee Waltz, and for those familiar with the song, that's exactly what happened. I "Tennessee Waltzed" that girl clean away from her boyfriend. In his defense, there was nothing he could do (refer to back cover) and if you could see my wife you'd know there was nothing else I could do but to marry her.

Much to everyone's shock, on September 5th 1959 we eloped. The Justice of the Peace was a local mechanic who was good at multitasking. Our witnesses were his elderly neighbors—one of them dozed off during the ceremony. Maybe I should have worn lime green to keep them awake! Our elopement caused us to miss my father's birthday celebration, which angered my family until I proceeded to provide the best excuse ever. So, if I'm late or running behind schedule, don't be quick to anger or jump to conclusions because as history has shown, I probably have the very best reason. In fact, in my house, if someone's late, even if by a mere few minutes, we say, "What are doing, marrying someone?" And I can tell you that if you're late, you'd better be...

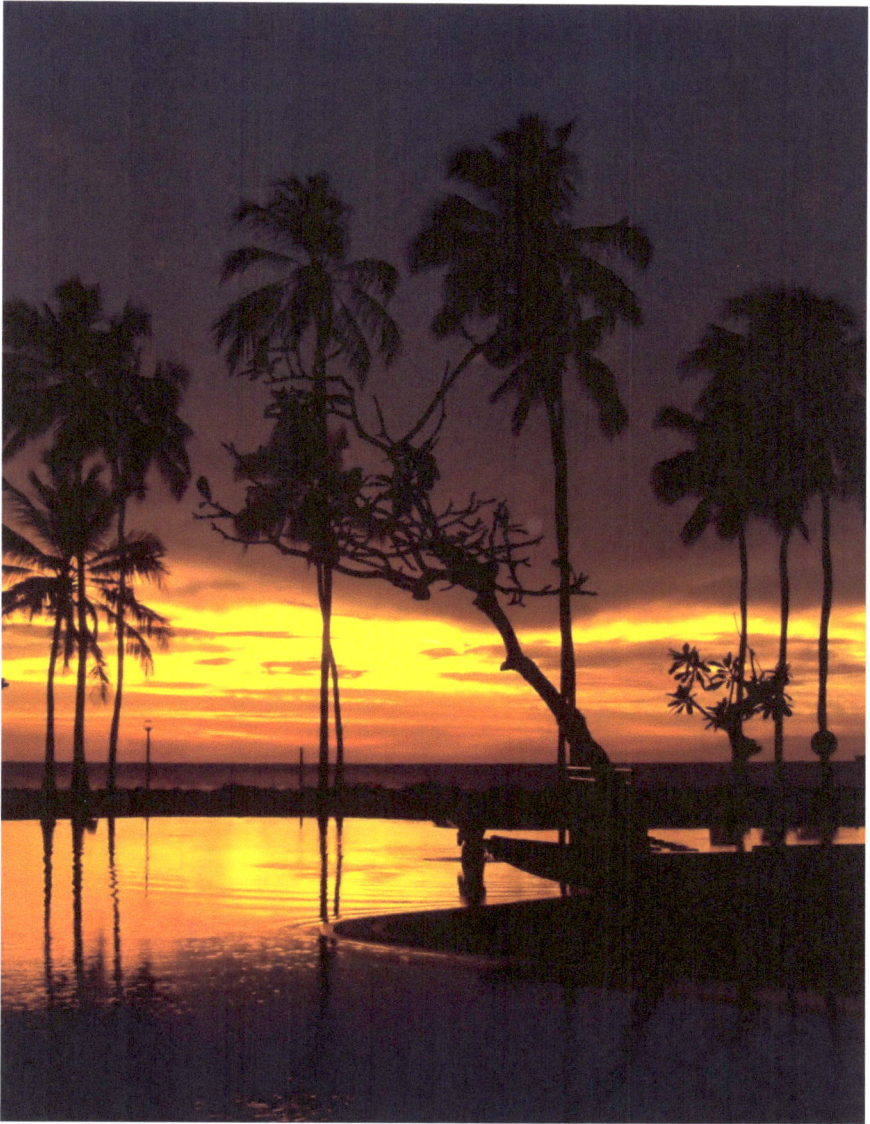

Sunset
End of a Positive Day

Because of the support of so many, because of the advanced medical care I received, because of my family, I live the life I knew before cancer. If you'd like to see for yourself, come find me on the golf course. You can't miss me. I'm the handsome man whose pants don't fit. You see, I'm doing so well that I've gained some weight, which is quite a feat for a Pozza. Usually, all we have to do is stand in one place long enough and the pounds start melting off. Anyway, I thought about losing the new found pounds when a friend quickly advised me to keep the pounds and simply shop for new pants, but was certain to add that I wasn't to shop alone. Message received. I can beat cancer four times, but can't be trusted to buy my own pants. As I said, I'm back to my life before cancer. Other than that, I look the same. At one point during treatment, my hair started to thin. I thought a baseball cap would hide that fact nicely, while looking sporty at the same time. My wife thought that a fedora would be more stylish and hide it better. That's code for her opinion that baseball caps look sloppy. It was the age old sporty vs. sloppy debate. But, as luck would have it, just as I had her in the grip of reason, my hair came back the same as it was before. (One more time, refer to back cover.)

As I look back over my life, I think of my time spent serving our country in the United States Air Force. I was a member of the Strategic Air Command and learned to develop a positive attitude. I feel the training I received during that part of my life was critical in helping me get through many things, including my cancer treatments.

Being a cancer survivor becomes part of your identity. I don't resist that fact, but embrace it. I take pride in the fact that I beat it. I beat it like a drum. Beat it with a stick. Beat it to the punch. It hasn't weakened me, but has rather strengthened my resolve. I feel I am the luckiest man on Earth. One reason for writing this is to inform patients, their families, and their friends that treatments are forever evolving and survival rates are climbing higher and higher. I realize that cancer will continue to claim the lives of loved ones, but the chances of surviving and living are better than ever and will be even more so tomorrow. Advances in medicine and technology are on your side. Make sure you believe it. I believe it because as I write this account, my CT scan results boast my remission. My treatments ended in November of 2012. Six months later, after a few follow-up visits, my doctor determined that I was in remission. I've been for almost two years now and I thank God every day.

With that, I'd like to take this opportunity to thank my family and friends for believing right alongside me. I want to thank the people who prayed for me, without even knowing me. I want to thank my doctors, nurses, and the Dyson Center staff for treating the person and not just the disease—allowing their expertise to intersect with compassion and personal attention.

Regrettably, I cannot bottle my DNA as I made light of at the start, but I can provide this short account. I can tally my flaws and strengths, my triumphs and missteps for all to read, simply, or not so simply, because I am here to do so.

So where do I go from here? In short, I intend to live to age 90 or older, and I'll not let prostate cancer, skin cancer, melanoma, lung cancer, tricky garage doors, or freakishly aggressive chickens get in my way. I'm Nick Pozza, a four-time cancer survivor, and forever, the leader of the band.

The End

www.ingramcontent.com/pod-product-compliance
Lightning Source LLC
Chambersburg PA
CBHW041304290326
41931CB00032B/37